FIBROMYALGIA
MAKING SENSE OF IT

By

Steven & Lorna Carroll

First Edition

ISBN 978-1-365-70090-3

Table of Contents

PAGE

What Is Fibromyalgia?   5

Possible Causes Of Fibromyalgia   7

Who Does Fibromyalgia Affect?   10

Risk Factors For Fibromyalgia   12

Is Fibromyalgia Real?   15

Symptoms Of Fibromyalgia   17

Diagnostic Criteria For Fibromyalgia   26

Treatment Options   34

Alternative Medicine   55

Living With Chronic Pain   56

20 Tips For Dealing With Fibromyalgia   59

Improving Your Quality Of Life   62

What Is Fibromyalgia?

Fibromyalgia is a poorly understood medical disorder that involves the experience of widespread pain in the muscles, joints, and tissues along with extra-musculoskeletal symptoms of sleep disturbances, memory problems, chronic fatigue, and issues related to mood.

There has been much research on this disorder. While the exact cause of fibromyalgia is unknown, most researchers feel that fibromyalgia takes painful sensations experienced by the sufferer and amplifies them in the brain, resulting in the sensation of pain with even light touch.

In a sense, fibromyalgia is believed to be a brain disorder caused by abnormal processing of pain signals by the brain.

- Fibromyalgia generally develops after a person has experienced some kind of physical trauma or has had surgery.
- Others develop the disorder following a great psychological stressor or following a minor infection.
- Still others do not have a dramatic shift from normal health to having fibromyalgia but instead have the symptoms develop gradually with no identifiable event causing the disease.

For reasons that are not completely clear, women have a greater chance of developing fibromyalgia when compared to men. Interestingly, those who have fibromyalgia also have a greater incidence of temporomandibular joint disorders (TMJ disease), tension-type headaches, depression, irritable bowel syndrome, and anxiety disorders.

Fibromyalgia has no known cure although sufferers have used various types of medications to make the symptoms more tolerable. Non-medical therapies for fibromyalgia include reducing stress levels, relaxation, exercise, acupuncture, nutritional supplementation, and other alternative therapies.

Possible Causes Of Fibromyalgia

There is no general consensus as to what causes fibromyalgia. Many doctors speculate that there isn't a single cause to the disorder but that it involves several different physical and emotional factors that work together to cause the disease.

These are some things that may be related to who gets fibromyalgia and who does not:

- **Genetic factors.** There may be some yet unknown genetic reasons why some people get fibromyalgia and others do not. It is known to run in families although it does not appear that there is a single gene involved in getting fibromyalgia. Genetic mutations have not yet been discovered but may play a role in developing the disease. According to the National Institute of Arthritis, Musculoskeletal, and Skin diseases, there may be genes in the human genome that regulate the ways the body handles pain. Those who have fibromyalgia may have inherited genes that result in an exaggerated response to pain in situations that another individual would not find painful.

- **Hormones.** Fibromyalgia occurs to a much greater degree in women when compared to men. There may be something about female hormones that trigger the disease in women but not in men. The hormonal milieu in women is much different in women than it is in men and the presence of female hormones may affect the nerves in such a way as to make fibromyalgia more likely.

- **Certain infections.** Because fibromyalgia can develop following an infection, it has been speculated that certain types of infections make fibromyalgia worse or trigger the onset of the disease in susceptible individuals.

- **Emotional Trauma.** People with post-traumatic stress disorder from childhood or other types of trauma are at a greater risk of developing fibromyalgia. Exactly how psychic trauma can lead to the physical manifestations of fibromyalgia is not yet clear.

- **Stress.** People who experience greater levels of stress in their lives have a greater incidence of fibromyalgia. Whether it is from a single stressor or multiple stressors over the course of a lifetime that contributes to fibromyalgia is not yet clear.

- **Brain chemicals.** Some researchers are looking into the idea that low levels of serotonin and other brain neurotransmitters affect the way the brain responds to pain. Additionally, there may be increased levels of substance P, the neurochemical that results in the sensation of pain. Finally, there may be lower levels of endogenous endorphins, the brain chemicals that protect us from the experience of pain, in patients suffering from fibromyalgia.

- **Trauma to the brain and spinal cord.** Some research has pointed to the idea that a sudden trauma to the spinal cord and brain trigger a decreased ability to respond to pain sensations in a normal way.

- **Sleep difficulties.** People with fibromyalgia commonly suffer from disorders of sleep. Whether the sleep problems cause the fibromyalgia or are the result of fibromyalgia is not yet clear. Poor sleep habits have been known to alter the levels of certain brain chemicals that contribute to fibromyalgia.

Who Does Fibromyalgia Affect?

At any given point in time, 2% of the American population is said to suffer from fibromyalgia, an estimated 5 million adults, or 1 in 50 people. Women are more highly affected than men are. In fact, 3.4% of women have the disorder compared to only 0.5% of men.

This means that the male to female ratio comparing women with fibromyalgia and men with the disease is about 7:1. It also means that 80 to 90% of all fibromyalgia sufferers are women although 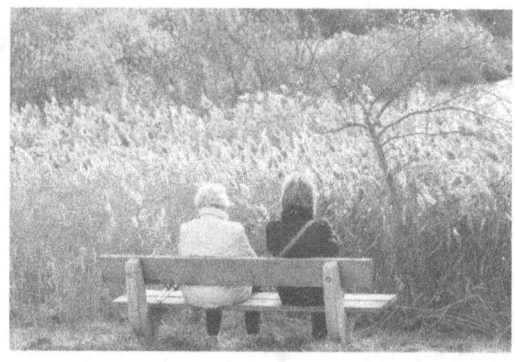 men and children also suffer from fibromyalgia.

Most people get the diagnosis of fibromyalgia during their middle-aged years. The overall prevalence of fibromyalgia increases with age. Fibromyalgia is the second most common musculoskeletal disorder behind osteoarthritis.

As mentioned, the diagnosis of fibromyalgia increases with age. 60% of fibromyalgia patients receive their diagnosis in their 30s and 40s, while another 35% will receive the diagnosis in their 20s or when they are between the ages of 50 and 65. It is rare to have a first time diagnosis of fibromyalgia under the age of 20 or over the age of 65.

As for women of working age who were hospitalized with a diagnosis of fibromyalgia, those with fibromyalgia were nearly ten times less likely to return to the workforce and four times less likely to be hired for another job within one year following the hospitalization when compared to those hospitalized for other musculoskeletal disorders.

For men and women who work with fibromyalgia, those with the disease miss about 17 days of work each year when compared to missing only 6 days per year for those who do not have fibromyalgia. The diagnosis of fibromyalgia is associated with lesser levels of health-associated quality of life and a decrease in work productivity.

Fibromyalgia appears to be related to other types of rheumatic disease. Those diagnosed with fibromyalgia also suffered from diseases like rheumatoid arthritis and systemic lupus erythematosus about 25 to 65% of the time.

Risk Factors For Fibromyalgia

Certain people carry more risk factors for getting fibromyalgia than others. Some of these risk factors include the following:

- **Family history.** If you have a close relative with fibromyalgia, you have an increased chance of getting the disorder as well. Unlike many genetic diseases, however, the links between who gets fibromyalgia in your family and who doesn't isn't based on the usual genetic principles. This means that just about any kind of relationship can exist between you and the other relative you have who has fibromyalgia.

- **Gender.** Women have an increased risk of being diagnosed with fibromyalgia when compared to men. This may be due to hormonal influences or to gender differences we do not yet understand.

- **History of a rheumatic disease.** If you suffer from a rheumatic disease such as SLE (lupus) or rheumatoid arthritis, you also stand a greater chance of being diagnosed with fibromyalgia. It is still possible to get fibromyalgia without any of these diseases or any other type of autoimmune disease. As far as research has shown, fibromyalgia itself is not an autoimmune disease.

- **Menopause.** Women are more likely to be diagnosed with fibromyalgia around the time of menopause.

This could mean that fibromyalgia is related to the sudden loss of estrogen associated with the coming of menopause.

- **Lack of physical conditioning.** Most women with fibromyalgia do not partake in a program of regular exercise, although it does afflict some women who have been active throughout their lives.

- **Surgery.** Some cases of fibromyalgia have been associated with having surgery in the not too distant past. The exact relationship between surgery and getting fibromyalgia, however, has not been made clear.

- **Spinal cord or brain trauma.** Some women develop fibromyalgia after a significant injury or accident that may or may not have set up the right biochemical conditions in the brain for getting fibromyalgia.

- **Stress.** Some people with fibromyalgia develop fibromyalgia after a major psychological stressor. Exactly how stress predisposes a person to fibromyalgia, however, is not completely clear.

- **Having insomnia.** While it is known that people with fibromyalgia do not sleep well, it is not known whether or not a lack of sleep is a risk factor for getting fibromyalgia or if lack of sleep stems from already having fibromyalgia. A lack of sleep is known to decrease a person's level of brain serotonin, which increases the sensitivity to pain. In some research studies, women have been deprived of sleep and have gotten symptoms similar to fibromyalgia.

- **Depression.** Women with depression have a higher risk of also having the diagnosis of fibromyalgia. The two diseases may stem from the same thing—low levels of brain serotonin.

Is Fibromyalgia Real?

It is difficult to know whether a particular disease is real when there are no x-rays or lab tests that fully identify the disease. This is the case in fibromyalgia. For this reason, doctors and researchers have come up with strict criteria that help identify whether or not a person has fibromyalgia, as it is one of the most difficult conditions to diagnose.

People with fibromyalgia must have a certain number of trigger point sensitivities in various body areas, which will be described later. This is involves doing a particular exam that assesses the patient's pain when touching specific body areas. If there are enough trigger points deemed sensitive and if the person has the other non-pain symptoms related to fibromyalgia it is said that they meet the criteria for having fibromyalgia.

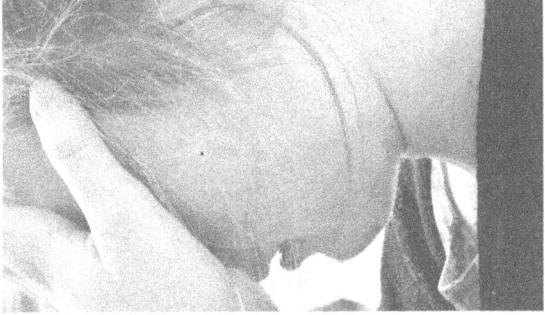

In a sense, fibromyalgia is no different from diagnosing most mental disorders. In mental disorders, there are no hard findings on labs and x-rays to identify the diseases and yet, when certain criteria are met, the individual is said to have the disorder. Like mental disorders for which there is no hard data to prove their existence, fibromyalgia is real. With the help of a careful history and specialized physical examination, the diagnosis of fibromyalgia can be confidently made.

If you believe you have fibromyalgia, make sure you see a doctor who can perform the specified physical examinations.

If you pass the criteria for fibromyalgia, then you have the disease.

Symptoms Of Fibromyalgia

Fibromyalgia is not just about muscle pain. There are many different symptoms of fibromyalgia. It is not necessary to have every symptom listed below in order to have the disease.

Some common symptoms of fibromyalgia include the following:

- **Chronic pain in the muscles associated with tightness in the muscles and muscle spasm.** Chronic musculoskeletal pain is the most characteristic symptom seen in almost everyone who has fibromyalgia. This is what usually causes the individual to seek medical attention in the first place. Fibromyalgia pain is widespread, felt in almost all body areas. It is often described as throbbing, aching, or dull pain although it can consist of deeply sharp pains as well. The pain is usually felt in the muscles and soft tissues of the body and will come and go in an irregular pattern. Some people have pain throughout their entire body.

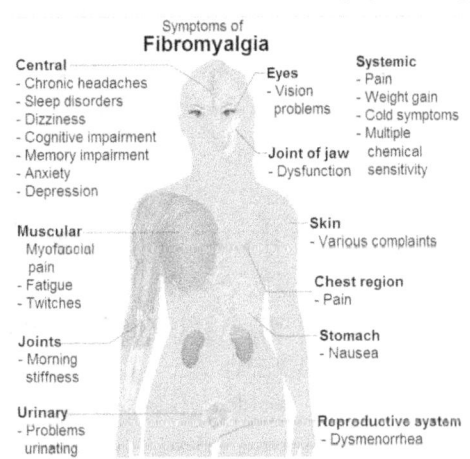

Symptoms of
Fibromyalgia

Central
- Chronic headaches
- Sleep disorders
- Dizziness
- Cognitive impairment
- Memory impairment
- Anxiety
- Depression

Muscular
  Myofascial pain
- Fatigue
- Twitches

Joints
- Morning stiffness

Urinary
- Problems urinating

Eyes
- Vision problems

Joint of jaw
- Dysfunction

Systemic
- Pain
- Weight gain
- Cold symptoms
- Multiple chemical sensitivity

Skin
- Various complaints

Chest region
- Pain

Stomach
- Nausea

Reproductive system
- Dysmenorrhea

- **Tender points in the body.** Besides the intense muscle soreness and aching of the body, those with

Fibromyalgia have localized areas of the body, usually near joints, that are extremely tender to the touch, especially when pushed on with the fingers. This pain is not associated with pain in the joints themselves but is found in the soft tissue that surrounds the joints, including the tendons and ligaments. The tender points are usually superficial in location, near the skin's surface. They are also not randomly occurring tender points but are in predictable areas of the body as evidenced by the exam, which will be elucidated below. Pressure on these specific tender points can result in extreme pain.

- **Fatigue, which can be moderate or severe, associated with decreased energy levels.** Fatigue is the second most common complaint in fibromyalgia after pain symptoms. The fatigue tends to linger and be unassociated with the amount of rest or sleep the person gets. Some with fibromyalgia feel as though the fatigue reminds them of the type of fatigue experienced when one had the flu. Others say it feels as though the fatigue is similar to the fatigue experienced when working too long after getting insufficient sleep. The fatigue is worse when getting up in the morning and occurs after a minimum amount of activity, such as house cleaning or shopping for groceries. People with fibromyalgia are too tired to exercise or to engage in sex. They tend to be too tired to start on a project, even something they otherwise would look forward to. They are often too tired to sustain an adequate amount of productivity at work.

- **Insomnia or the inability to get an adequate amount of sleep.** They often feel just as fatigued upon arising as they did when going to sleep. There may be difficulty getting to sleep in the first place associated with sleep that is easily disturbed, light, and uncomfortable. In the morning, they may feel as though they had unrefreshing sleep and may feel exhausted. The lack of sleep contributes to the chronic fatigue the fibromyalgia sufferers often experience.

There are actual EEG changes experienced when fibromyalgia sufferers are sleeping. They have EEG changes that mimic the awake state, even as the fibromyalgia sufferer appears to be sleeping. The EEG changes associated with deep sleep are somewhat lacking when a person with fibromyalgia is sleeping, limiting the amount of time the individual spends in the deepest stages of sleep. This means that the body cannot rejuvenate itself and the sufferer feels tired in the morning.

- **Muscle stiffness after waking up or when remaining in one position for a long period of time.** Research has shown that many people with fibromyalgia feel stiff in the morning when they first get up. The stiffness extends to include the arms, legs, and back, giving the sufferer the feeling that they need to loosen up their muscles before being able to go about their regular daily activities.

The stiffness may persist for only a few minutes after arising or can last up to twenty minutes after getting out of bed in the morning. People with severe fibromyalgia feel stiff all the time and no amount of relaxation or stretching appears to relieve the muscle stiffness.

The type of stiffness experienced by those with fibromyalgia is different from the minor aching and muscle stiffness many people feel after a restless night of sleep. Rather, it is stiffness that is typical of those who have inflammatory arthritis or rheumatoid arthritis, which is difficult to get rid of.

- **Problems with memory, concentration, and the performance of basic mental tasks.** This is often referred to as having "fibro fog" and interferes with the fibromyalgia sufferer's ability to be productive at work. Tasks take longer to accomplish and memory difficulties make it difficult to memorize the various steps of a given task given to the individual. Poor concentration can be profound so that the individual finds it difficult to get anything accomplished.

- **Depressive symptoms.** People with fibromyalgia often complain of symptoms consistent with depression. In fact, nearly half of all people who have fibromyalgia already have the diagnosis of depression or an anxiety disorder at the time they are diagnosed with fibromyalgia syndrome.

Researchers aren't sure whether or not the stress associated with constant fatigue and ongoing pain causes an anxiety state seen in fibromyalgia. It is also possible that the pain from fibromyalgia results in less activity and an increase in social withdrawal that can lead to depressive symptoms.

Depression, whether it predates the diagnosis of fibromyalgia or occurs after the person has been diagnosed with fibromyalgia, may be a part of the syndrome itself and may be related to brain changes common in the two diseases. The same is true with anxiety, which may be an actual part of the disease of fibromyalgia itself.

- **Swelling and tingling of the hands.** Fibromyalgia sufferers often exhibit neurological complaints, including burning pain, tingling, and numbness of the hands. No one knows the cause of these neurological complaints even though they are very common in those who have fibromyalgia. These sensations, known as paresthesia, seem to occur at the same time a fibromyalgia sufferer experiences stiffness in the morning, although some people have paresthesia symptoms lasting most of the day.

- **Chronic headaches.** People with fibromyalgia are more prone to migraine or tension headaches than those who do not have fibromyalgia. Up to 70 percent of all fibromyalgia, patients also complain of chronic headaches.

The headaches are often related to the chronic pain in the upper aspect of the back and the neck in those who have fibromyalgia. This type of pain leads to inflammation of the scalp muscles, which is the cause of tension headaches (muscle-contraction headaches).

There are also trigger points in the back of the head and neck, which can lead to muscle contraction headaches.

Even though headaches are often associated with fibromyalgia, any chronic headache condition should be evaluated by a physician to make sure the headaches are solely related to fibromyalgia and not to some other condition or disease.

- **Irritable bowel syndrome symptoms.** People with fibromyalgia often complain of nausea, bloating, abdominal pain, and constipation. Some have constipation alternating with diarrhea, which is a typical symptom of irritable bowel syndrome. These gastrointestinal symptoms are found in about 40-70 percent of fibromyalgia patients. They often complain of indigestion, acid reflux, or GERD, which stands for "gastroesophageal reflux disease."

- **Facial and jaw tenderness.** People with fibromyalgia can have pain in the temporomandibular joints or across the facial muscles. Some patients will meet the criteria for having temporomandibular joint disease (TMJ) along with the criteria for fibromyalgia.

- **Oversensitivity to stimuli.** Those with fibromyalgia will complain of oversensitivity to certain odors, bright lights, loud noises, cold air, certain foods, or medications. They may be intolerant to another's perfume or find themselves only comfortable in a warm, dark, and quiet place. This limits the fibromyalgia patient's ability to participate in many areas of normal daily activities.

- **Irritable bladder symptoms.** Fibromyalgia patients often find themselves with an increase in urinary frequency an urgency. They may feel as though they have a bladder infection when the ordinary tests used to diagnose bladder infections are negative for infection. They may have difficulty getting to the restroom in time, leading to urinary urge incontinence. Unfortunately, medications for urinary urge incontinence often exacerbate symptoms of constipation so these medications are often not indicated in those fibromyalgia patients with irritable bowel syndrome symptoms.

- **Increased menstrual cramps.** Women with fibromyalgia who are also within childbearing age often complain of severe menstrual cramps and heavy vaginal flow. These menstrual symptoms are often long lasting—occurring up until the time of menopause. When menopause occurs, they often have a greater number and intensity of hot flashes and night sweats when compared to those who do not have fibromyalgia.

- **Decreased tolerance for exercise.** Fibromyalgia patients often do not tolerate the rigors of exercise, many complaining of increased pain in the muscles following exercise. Even though you will see that exercise is effective in the management of fibromyalgia, it is often difficult to get started in an exercise program when the patient feels as though the exercise will worsen their symptoms.

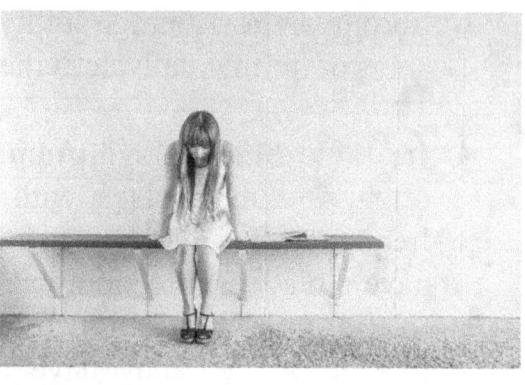

- **A sensation of swelling of the feet and hands.** Fibromyalgia patients often feel as though their hands and feet are swollen although, to physical appearances, no swelling can be detected.

- **Symptoms of restless legs syndrome.** Restless legs syndrome is a condition where the legs feel very uncomfortable and only experience relief of these symptoms when the legs are moved or shaken. The individual ends up tossing and turning, especially at night because keeping the legs still is an intolerable feeling.

  Fibromyalgia patients often feel symptoms of restless leg syndrome, which may worsen at nighttime or when the patient is trying to sleep. This can exacerbate the insomnia symptoms typical in those who have fibromyalgia.

- **Factors That Affect Symptoms**

➤ The symptoms of fibromyalgia tend to fluctuate according to various internal and external conditions.

➤ Fibromyalgia symptoms are different throughout the

24

course of the day. Shortly after getting out of bed in the morning, the late afternoon period, and the evening are usually times when fibromyalgia symptoms are the most severe.

➢ Symptoms tend to worsen under conditions of increased fatigue and stress/tension.

➢ Symptoms can worsen with inactivity, which is why regular movement and low impact exercise is so important.

➢ Colder months, or when the indoor air becomes drafty can make pain worse.

➢ Overexertion tends to make the symptoms worse.

➢ Hormonal changes affect symptoms.

➢ Many female fibromyalgia patients feel worsened symptoms in the premenstrual phase and during the time of menopause.

➢ Emotional factors such as anxiety and depression tend to exacerbate the pain experienced by those who suffer from fibromyalgia.

Diagnostic Criteria For Fibromyalgia

Because fibromyalgia has no blood test or x-ray used to make the diagnosis, the American College of Rheumatology has set forth guidelines for the diagnosis of the condition. Fibromyalgia can mimic other diseases, including Lyme disease, HIV disease, degenerative spine diseases, low thyroid conditions, and certain types of cancer.

While there are blood tests and other testing modalities for these types of diseases, these can take time and a simple diagnostic examination can set the record straight as to whether or not you have fibromyalgia.

The latest criteria set for the diagnosis of fibromyalgia were developed in 2010. According to the guidelines set up by the American College of Rheumatology, you are suffering from fibromyalgia if you meet the following criteria:

- You have the experience of nearly constant pain on all four quadrants of your body. This includes having pain on both sides of the body as well as pain localized above and below the level of the waist.

- You have the experience of tenderness in at least 11 of the 18 listed tender points exhibited by people who have fibromyalgia.

This diagnostic protocol has its critics. Because the symptoms of fibromyalgia tend to wax and wane, an individual who does not meet the criteria for fibromyalgia on one evaluation may meet the criteria for the disease at a later time, even though it may be only a few hours later.

The criteria are also mainly pain-related and ignore the many other symptoms associated with fibromyalgia, including the fatigue symptoms, depressive symptoms, gastrointestinal symptoms, and urinary tract complaints.

The WPI

The 2010 diagnostic criteria for fibromyalgia lessened the role of trigger point tenderness in the diagnosis of fibromyalgia even though many doctors still use this as a factor in making the diagnosis.

Instead of trigger point tenderness, the American College of Rheumatology proposed the use of the widespread pain index, also known as the WPI. The WPI used a checklist involving nineteen areas of the human body.

With the WPI, the patient gives a positive checkmark if they experienced pain in a particular area within the previous seven days. Nineteen different areas of the body are included so that a given patient could have a score of between 0 and 19.

In addition, the severity of the various symptoms in four different categories that are not related to pain, such as mental symptoms, urinary tract symptoms, and gastrointestinal symptoms are taken into consideration. These areas are scored on a scale from zero to three so that the total possible score in this section is 12. This part of the evaluation is called the symptom severity score or SS. Both the WPI and the SS are taken into account when making the diagnosis of fibromyalgia.

The Trigger Point Evaluation

Your doctor may evaluate your fibromyalgia using the trigger point evaluation, also called the tender point evaluation. Even though the use of this examination has been minimized by the latest recommendations, many doctors still feel that the evaluation of these trigger points are an important part of the evaluation.

When you have a trigger point evaluation, the doctor will press on each area with a single fingertip. The amount of pressure used is just enough to cause the nail bed to whiten. The doctor will then ask you if you feel pain to the touch.

Pain Points Seen In Fibromyalgia:

- The area between your shoulder blades

- The very top part of your shoulders

- The back part of the head

- The front part of the neck

- The upper chest area

- The inside soft area of the elbows

- The upper hip area

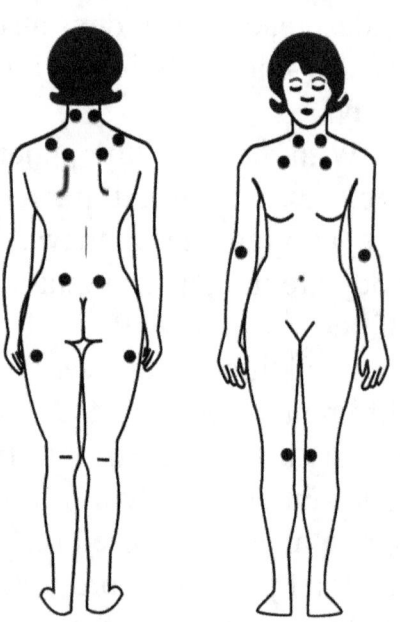

- The inner knees
- The sides of the hip joints

Because other conditions yield symptoms that can mimic fibromyalgia, the doctor will often rule these out in order to make sure that the diagnosis is fibromyalgia and not some other disease. This can involve blood tests used to identify conditions such as hypothyroidism, HIV disease, Lyme disease, and rheumatoid arthritis.

Tests you might undergo besides blood tests include x-ray evaluations, CT scans of the body, and MRI scans to look for spinal degenerative disease or possibly cancer. Some doctors do tissue biopsies for cancer along with sleep study evaluations and psychological evaluations.

It can help the doctor if you keep a diary of the symptoms you are experiencing. Such a diary might include:

- Where your pain is located
- What your pain is like
- The severity of your pain
- How long the pain lasts
- Other non-pain related symptoms

Keeping this diary can help the doctor get a personalized picture of your daily symptoms and may help make the diagnosis of fibromyalgia.

Fibromyalgia Pain Points

As previously mentioned, fibromyalgia is generally difficult to diagnose, it can mimic other diseases, including

Lyme disease, HIV disease, degenerative spine diseases, low thyroid conditions, and certain types of cancer, and it is really a matter of ruling out these types of conditions.

According to the American College of Rheumatology, a diagnosis of fibromyalgia requires the experience of nearly constant pain on all four quadrants of your body. This includes having pain on both sides of the body as well as pain localized above and below the level of the waist. Additionally, the criterion requires tenderness in at least 11 of the 18 listed tender points exhibited by people who have fibromyalgia.

Tender Points

- **The Neck** - The back of your neck is considered to contain major points of pain. The tender points could be at the base of the skull or where your shoulders meet your neck and anywhere in between. With the neck area, there is also a strong likelihood of referred pain, which means the real area of pain is causing pressure on nerves. This will result in a sensation of pain in a seemingly unrelated area. Your doctor will probably check for various related points in the neck muscles.

  The front area of the neck is also strongly related to pain, so the whole neck can become very painful in this condition. The muscular points of pain at the front of the neck are the big muscles at the sides of your head. These are called the sternocleidomastoid muscles and are involved with a wide range of neck movements. This is one of the major reasons fibromyalgia causes such intense neck pain, possibly frequent headaches and sleep problems.

- **The Elbow -** Elbow pain also seems to be common in fibromyalgia. Keep in mind this is also a common site of injuries. Just because your elbows are aching doesn't mean you have the condition in question. If you do a lot of lifting and twisting motions with your arms on a regular basis, this can cause a condition known as tendonitis and the elbows are a common area for this type of injury. With fibromyalgia, the elbow pain will be persistent and usually felt on the outside and the center of the arm.

- **Hips -** The hips are another major pain point in fibromyalgia. Hip pain is also often of major concern when it comes to osteoarthritis and rheumatoid arthritis. Fibromyalgia pain in this area is not felt in the joints. Instead, it is centered in the gluteus maximus and gluteus minor muscles. What does this mean in plain English? It means your butt muscles hurt most of the time. Sitting can become excruciating and standing may also hurt at times. Pain in the butt is a major contributor to sleep problems associated with fibromyalgia.

- **Lower Back -** As if hip pain were not enough to deal with, the next major point is the lower back. There are multitudes of physical problems, which can cause lower back pain. Sitting for lengthy periods can cause pain here. Standing too much can also do the same. A lack of exercise and being overweight can cause this pain. Injuries are a culprit too. How is it experienced when people are dealing with fibromyalgia? How is it different? There are usually two distinct trigger points right at the top of those butt muscles. Even gentle pressure on these little indentations above the hips will induce severe pain.

- **The Knees** - The knees hurt and this is another point, which requires some clarification yet is usually involved with fibromyalgia points. There are many potential knee problems and your physician will most likely need to run some tests to determine if you might have an untreated injury or serious issues, which require different treatment. The distinct nature of fibromyalgia pain in the knees is that pain and sensitivity is focused on the back of the knees, on the soft side. Mechanically, this is a bundle of nerves and tendons related to the support of the buttocks and lower back. Are you starting to see the pattern?

- **Upper Back** - So far, all of these points of pain are related to bodily support muscles or muscles, which hold you up and make you functional in general life activities. The upper back is a point of fibromyalgia pain related to shoulder and neck support. Actual pressure points will be located between the spine and shoulder blades. This is the area we often see people rubbing in states of fatigue. The difference is, with fibromyalgia, these muscles called the trapezius muscles will hurt almost all of the time, contributing to neck pain, displacing the shoulders, and leading to balance issues and, ironically, neck pain.

- **Chest** - Chest muscles are checked for pain by doctors to make a diagnosis. Sudden chest pain is not the same as what is being described here. If you have sudden chest pain and / or shortness of breath, dial 911 or 999 immediately (or dial immediately whichever healthcare emergency number is relevant to your specific country). Any regular chest pain must be addressed by a physician. Otherwise, the pain with fibromyalgia will have focused pain on one or both sides of the sternum. The sternum is the long bone down the center of your chest, so the pain points would be close to this bone and all its connections to the ribs. In addition, the pain is localized, not connected with side chest muscles or breathing muscles.

You may not be counting a full eighteen points, but when you consider each of these points to be bilateral, occurring on both sides, you start to get an idea of how fibromyalgia pain can extend itself. In the neck, there are at least eight potential points alone.

The hips and lower back comprise four to six potential points. It is the distribution of pain along the planes of the body, which involve areas of focal balance. Neck, shoulders, lower back, hips, elbows, and knees.

Treatment Options

Once you have been given the diagnosis of fibromyalgia, you may be interested in what treatments are available. Because no one knows the exact cause of the disease, the treatments are completely empirical, based on what seems to help the symptoms and what makes sufferers feel better.

Medication

Many medications have been tried and are in use for the management of fibromyalgia symptoms, including sleeping medication, medications for pain, and antidepressant medications.

Some medications directly address the pain of fibromyalgia while others improve the mood related symptoms or help you sleep. You may have to try several different medications with your doctor's advice in order to find a single medication or 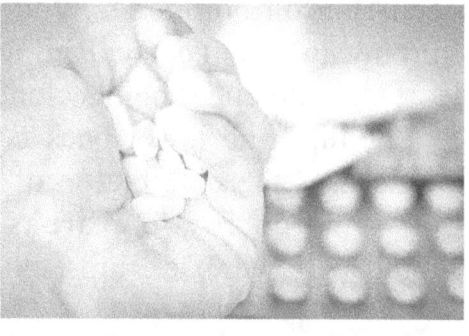 combination of medications that help manage the symptoms.

Medications that have been tried and used successfully in some fibromyalgia patients include the following:

- **Antidepressants.** These are among the first medications used to treat fibromyalgia. Antidepressants have been known to relieve symptoms of fatigue, improve pain symptoms, and improve one's ability to sleep. There are two types of medications used to treat fibromyalgia. The first includes the newer agents, such as selective serotonin reuptake inhibitors or SSRIs and the second include tricyclic antidepressants, which have been in use for many decades for the treatment of depression and many other related conditions.

- **Tricyclic Antidepressants.** These include medications such as nortriptyline (Pamelor) and amitriptyline. These act on the levels of neurotransmitters in the brain, specifically serotonin and norepinephrine. It is well known that people with chronic pain syndromes like fibromyalgia benefit by increasing these neurotransmitters in the brain. Tricyclic antidepressants have the ability to relax muscles that have become painful and elevate the effects of the body's natural endorphins, which are the innate painkillers of the brain. Tricyclic antidepressants work very well for people with fibromyalgia but have a variety of side effects than can be intolerable, including constipation, dry mouth, dry eyes, drowsiness, and dizziness.

- **SSRI Antidepressants.** As mentioned, these are a newer class of antidepressants that have effects on the fatigue, sleep problems, and pain exhibited by those with fibromyalgia. Of the many SSRI antidepressants available for use in people with fibromyalgia, three SSRIs have been studied the most. These include milnacipran (Savella), venlafaxine (Effexor), and duloxetine (Cymbalta). Of the three, both Cymbalta and Savella have received FDA approval for the management of fibromyalgia. Effexor has less medical research to support its effectiveness. Other SSRIs that have been studied for use in patients with fibromyalgia include fluoxetine (Prozac), citalopram (Celexa) and paroxetine (Paxil).

Antidepressants have different actions on the body. What works well for one individual with fibromyalgia may be ineffective for another individual with the disease. You may have to try more than one antidepressant or try antidepressants of different classes in order to find one that best controls the sleep problems, fatigue, and pain you are experiencing. Some doctors use more than one type of antidepressant at the same time so don't be alarmed if you are taking more than one.

- **Over-the-counter pain relievers.** Some people with fibromyalgia receive pain relief by taking acetaminophen. This has been known to increase the pain threshold so that pain is less significantly perceived. Other choices are nonsteroidal anti-inflammatory medication or NSAIDs, which include ibuprofen (marketed as Advil and Motrin) and naproxen (marketed as Naprosyn and Aleve). They act on pain and inflammation, reducing pain. The NSAIDs are not without side effects, which can include stomach upset, nausea, and stomach ulcers, especially with prolonged use. Things like bleeding in the stomach and heartburn can also be side effects of taking NSAID therapy, especially if you are over the age of 60 years. It is advisable to speak to your physician if you have to take NSAID therapy for more than ten days in a row. If you have a history of intestinal, stomach bleeding, or suffer from a bleeding disorder, make sure it is okay with your doctor to take these types of medications.

Acetaminophen has fewer side effects when compared to taking NSAID therapy but it cannot be taken safely by those who suffer from liver disease. In addition, if you take more than the recommended amount of acetaminophen, you run the risk of causing liver damage.

- **Muscle relaxants.** Some people with fibromyalgia have had relief of their muscle spasms by taking the drug cyclobenzaprine. This muscle relaxant has been found to lessen muscle tension and to help a person sleep better. Muscle relaxants act on the brain, which relaxes the muscles.

  Muscle relaxants, unfortunately, can have their own set of side effects. Some side effects of muscle relaxants you may notice include dizziness, dry mouth, blurry vision, unsteadiness, drowsiness, and an alteration in the color of the urine. Muscle relaxants also decrease the seizure threshold so they must be taken with caution in those who suffer from a seizure disorder. If muscle relaxants are taken by the elderly, they can increase the incidence of hallucinations and confusion.

- **Lyrica.** Also known as, pregabalin, Lyrica is the only FDA-approved drug for the treatment of fibromyalgia. It was initially marketed as an anti-seizure drug but was found to help those with fibromyalgia sleep better, have decreased pain and an improvement in fatigue.

- **Other anticonvulsant medications.** Gabapentin, marketed as Neurontin, is an anti-seizure medication that has been used on people with fibromyalgia with some success in relieving their pain.

- **Ultram.** Prescription pain-relievers have been used to manage the pain of fibromyalgia. One of them is Ultram (tramadol). It is a medication that is related to narcotics that acts on the brain to reduce the feelings of pain. It is sometimes used in the treatment of fibromyalgia because its addictive potential is less than that of narcotic pain relievers.

- **Benzodiazepines.** Benzodiazepines are commonly used medications in the management of anxiety disorders. Some of them include clonazepam (Klonopin), alprazolam (Xanax), lorazepam (Ativan) and diazepam (Valium). Besides acting on anxiety and sleep, they seem to help relax the muscle spasms of those who have fibromyalgia. They also help relieve the symptoms of restless legs syndrome, which is commonly associated with fibromyalgia. The biggest problem with benzodiazepines is that they are very addictive and it is all too easy to become physically dependent on these mediations. Some people use these medications in doses above the recommended amounts, resulting in adverse side effects.

- **Narcotic Pain Relievers.** Some people with fibromyalgia are prescribed narcotic pain relievers for the relief of their chronic pain. Some of these include oxycodone (OxyContin), hydrocodone (Lortab) and a combination of oxycodone and acetaminophen, marketed as Percocet. Hydrocodone and acetaminophen are sometimes used together in a medication called Vicodin. Because these medications are highly addictive, they should be used as a last resort for the treatment of fibromyalgia after the other medications have been tried without relief of the fibromyalgia symptoms. Close medical supervision is required if you decide to take these medications for your fibromyalgia.

Exercise

When fibromyalgia patients find themselves laid up in bed with chronic pain, the last thing they want to do is exercise. However, there is a lot of research to support that the right kind of exercise can actually reduce the pain of fibromyalgia and can help control the other symptoms as well.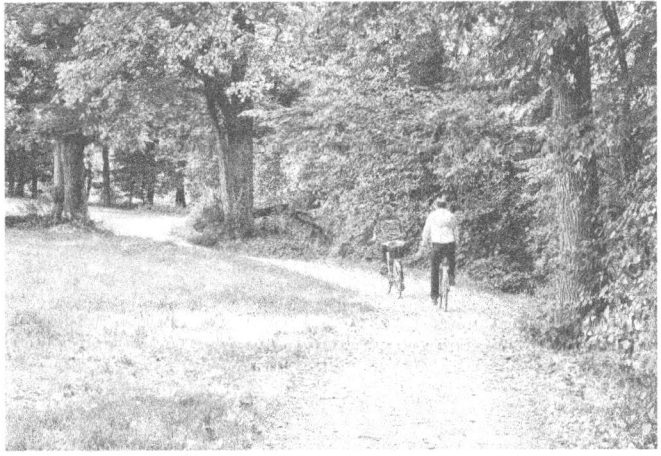

This doesn't mean you have to learn how to run a marathon. Here are some simple tips to help you begin to exercise so that you can eventually find relief of your symptoms.

- **Start exercising in bed if that's all you can do.** Begin by doing stretching exercises in bed. This will loosen up the muscles and help train your body to move better. Do this for about a half hour at a time, giving your body a chance to rest before trying again.

- **Recognize that it will be helpful.** Exercise is an extremely effective way to reduce the pain of fibromyalgia. It also improves your sleep and lessens the fatigue associated with fibromyalgia. Even though exercise seems to be the last thing you should be doing, you really need to believe that it can be helpful in controlling your symptoms.

- **Begin the process slowly.** When it comes to exercise, even if you didn't have fibromyalgia, the key is to begin slowly and work your way up to increasing levels of exercise. Try walking for five minutes every day and increase you're walking time by a minute or two every week until you find yourself able to exercise for up to 20-30 minutes per day. This may take a couple of months but gradually, you will find the exercise to be even easier. If the idea of "exercise" seems too hard, do things that increase the activity of the body such as getting around more on your feet, swimming, or using the stairs instead of the elevator. You don't have to begin a formal exercise program in order to be more active.

- **Pay attention to your body.** You need to listen to your body and tailor your exercise so that you don't overdo it. Some people try to do too much and end up becoming injured or 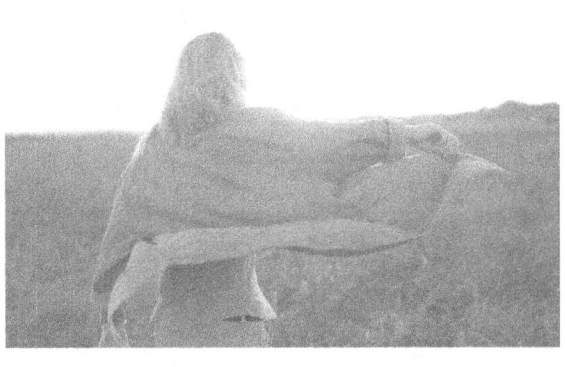 giving up too soon. Even if you were accustomed to being athletic before the diagnosis of fibromyalgia, things have changed and you have to recognize that things you could do before may currently be out of your reach. Practice with different levels of exercise until you find something that feels good to your body but does not injure you or worsen your pain.

- **Make an attempt every day.** Try not to skip any days when you have started exercising. If one exercise is boring to do every day, try to switch things up. Go swimming one day, take a walk the next, and use exercise equipment on another day. Warm pool exercises are very good for those with fibromyalgia and are less stressful on your joints. As swimming becomes easier, take your exercises to the ground and practice walking or using some kind of exercise equipment. Eventually, you will have a repertoire of things you can do that will make exercise fun and will allow you to do it on a daily basis. Try some different forms of exercise, such as Pilates, cycling, and strength training so that you never run out of things to do. Don't forget that exercise can be more fun if you have a buddy come along. Find a friend or family member to make your exercise routine more social and more fun.

- **Make modifications to your workout.** As a person with fibromyalgia, you need to take steps to avoid worsening your pain or becoming injured. This might mean planning your exercise to occur when your body feels at its best, which is usually between 10:00 am and 3:00 pm in people with 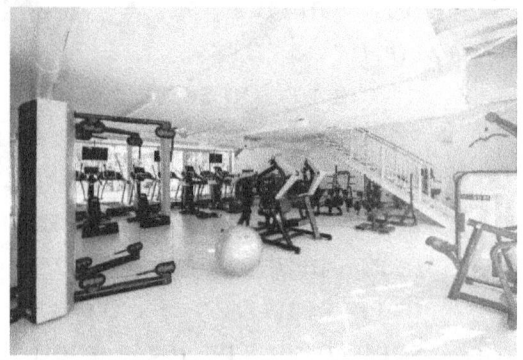 fibromyalgia. Be sure to stretch out before doing anything strenuous so you don't injury your muscles. Stretching can be done in a shower or in a warm bath, particularly if the muscles are very stiff. Try to exercise carefully, walking on flat surfaces, and avoiding uneven terrain. This will decrease your chances of tripping and falling, and will make your exercise go smoother.

- **Be careful with strength training as lifting heavy weights can contribute to injury.** Think about doing strength training with elastic bands and don't do multiple sets of the same exercise until a single set becomes easy and you have rested your muscles well between sets.

- **Take as many breaks as you need to in order to get the exercise done without wearing yourself out.** The biggest mistake you can make is to push through an exercise program when your body is telling you to rest. This only leads to injury or to feelings that exercise is too much for you so that you give up before you have reaped the benefits of exercise in the management of your fibromyalgia.

- **Do easy stretches after your exercise is over with and treat yourself to a bath or hot shower after your exercise is over with.** This will ease any tension left in the muscles and will reward you for a job well done.

- **Be patient with yourself.** You will not feel good about exercise the first few times you make an attempt at it. Try to pace yourself according to your level of pain and your energy level so that each episode of exercising leads to a positive end. Start exercising as slowly as you need to in order to begin to do something headed in the right direction

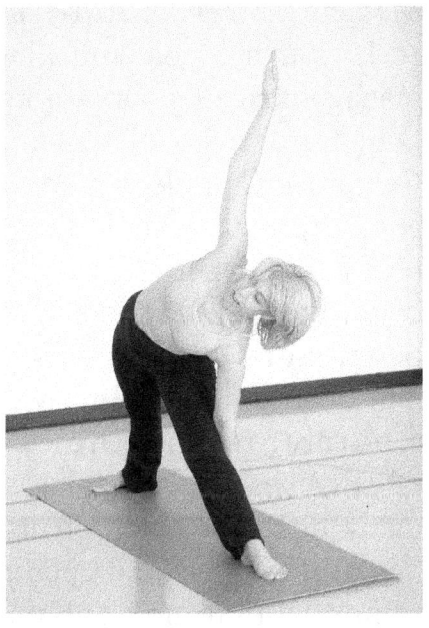

when it comes to exercise. Set reasonable goals and don't be discouraged if you aren't running marathons by the end of a couple of weeks of exercise. Exercise in someone who has fibromyalgia has to be done in baby steps so that you can enjoy exercise and find it to be beneficial as part of your newfound program of health and wellness.

Herbs And Supplements

Many people with fibromyalgia also use elements of alternative medicine to help control their symptoms. For many people, this includes taking supplements. There are several types of herbs and other supplements that can be used to control symptoms and maximize health. Common supplements used to help people with fibromyalgia include herbs obtained through the practices of Traditional Chinese Medicine, 5-HTP, SAM-e, and melatonin.

If you are contemplating using a supplement for the management of your fibromyalgia, make use of resources gotten from the National Center for Complementary and Alternative Medicine (NCCAM), which is an organization formed to better study supplements and other complementary treatments and their effectiveness in managing  many different kinds of disease states. Your doctor or an herbalist may also be good resources for you to try various remedies that may enhance your state of health with fibromyalgia.

There are some research studies available that indicate the effectiveness of certain herbal medicines and natural supplements in the treatment of fibromyalgia although there is not a lot of research on the subject. Fortunately, most supplements are completely harmless and are worth trying if your doctor feels it is okay to take them and you want to try something other than prescribed medications for the treatment of your fibromyalgia.

Here are some supplements that people have used to help control their fibromyalgia symptoms and that have some evidence of being beneficial:

- **5-Hydroxytryptophan.** This is also called 5-HTP and is one of the building blocks to making the neurotransmitter serotonin. Low levels of serotonin have been associated with depression and with those who have fibromyalgia. By taking 5-HTP, you may build your serotonin levels so that you can sleep better and have better resolution of your pain. Some studies have indicated that 5-HTP improves the amount of deep sleep that you get and can improve the symptoms of anxiety, insomnia, and depression that go along with having fibromyalgia.

  Most people have no problems taking 5-HTP. Unfortunately, some studies out of the late 1980s revealed that taking serotonin precursors such as 5-HTP and L-tryptophan was associated with the development of eosinophilia-myalgia syndrome, a serious medical condition that results in extreme muscle pain, burning rashes, and flu-like symptoms. For this reason, you should take 5-HTP with caution and discontinue taking it if you develop any of the symptoms noted above.

- **Melatonin.** Melatonin is a hormone produced naturally by the pineal gland near the brain that regulates a person's sleep-wake cycle. It is said to help a person feel sleepy when taken near bedtime so that sleep patterns can be restored to normal. There have been studies linking the taking of melatonin to pain reduction in those with fibromyalgia. It also improves sleep patterns and can be especially helpful in fibromyalgia patients who have difficulty sleeping and suffer from daytime fatigue.

  Melatonin is a natural hormone that is considered by most doctors to be completely safe. There are a few side effects to be concerned about. One note of caution: because melatonin can cause sleepiness during the day, it should be used at night and should not be taken by anyone who plans to take melatonin and operate a motor vehicle or use heavy equipment.

- **St. John's Wort.** There are no research studies on fibromyalgia and the taking of St. John's Wort indicating an effectiveness in taking the supplement. On the other hand, St. John's Wort 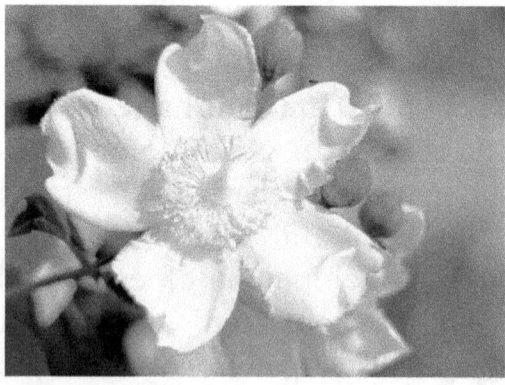 is very popular in Europe as a supplement in the management of depression. This means that fibromyalgia patients who also suffer from depressive symptoms may find relief in taking St. John's Wort.

Research on St. John's Wort and depression alone has revealed that St. John's Wort has better effectiveness when compared to placebo and works as well as some of the older antidepressants in the management of depression. Still other studies have compared St. John's Wort to modern SSRI medications for depression and have shown effectiveness of the supplement against these medications as well when it comes to managing depressive symptoms.

Most people tolerate taking St. John's Wort very well. Some common side effects to look out for are fatigue, skin rashes, and slight stomach upset. Remember not to take St. John's Wort with other types of antidepressants or even other supplements because certain combinations of the supplement and other medications or supplements can result in illness.

- **SAM-e.** SAM-e is a supplement that has equivocal findings when it comes to research studies on the supplement when taken by people with fibromyalgia. Some researchers believe that SAM-e can increase the level of dopamine and serotonin in the brain, improving mood and relieving depression. Other researchers are of the opinion that SAM-e increases the amount of restful sleep that a person can get. Still other research studies have shown no effectiveness of

SAM-e on any of these things. Most researchers feel that further studies are indicated in order to evaluate the effectiveness of SAM-e in relieving the various symptoms of fibromyalgia.

- **L Carnitine.** There are just a few research studies out there on the effectiveness of L carnitine on fibromyalgia symptoms. Some studies have demonstrated pain relief in those fibromyalgia patients that take L carnitine. In one particular study on L carnitine and fibromyalgia, 102 patients who suffered from fibromyalgia had improvements in their symptoms when they took L carnitine when compared to another group of individuals with fibromyalgia who took placebo medication. Because this study was not done on a very large sample of individuals, it was recommended that more studies be done to see if the same findings could be found when larger numbers of people were included in the study.

- **Probiotics.** Probiotics are natural dietary supplements that consist of live or encapsulated bacteria that are considered beneficial for digestive health. When taken in food containing probiotics or as probiotic supplements, it is felt that they replace bad bacteria in the gut so that the gut functions more smoothly without excess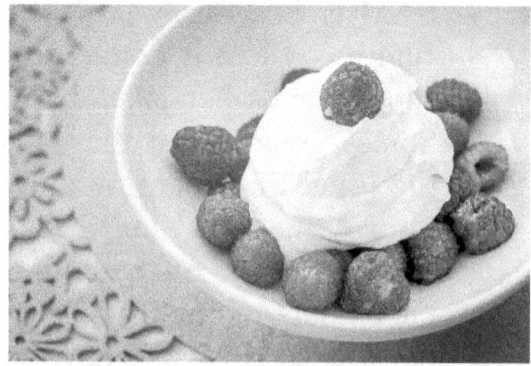

diarrhea, bloating, or constipation.

Probiotics are known to be helpful in those suffering from irritable bowel syndrome, which is a condition that many with fibromyalgia also have. Probiotics are felt to be beneficial in managing diarrhea, lessening the number of bowel infections or urinary tract infections a person has, and controlling symptoms of irritable bowel syndrome.

There can be mild side effects associated with taking probiotic supplements, including bloating or excess gas. Most people have no problems taking probiotics, however, and they should be tried in anyone with fibromyalgia and prominent symptoms of irritable bowel syndrome.

- **Miscellaneous Supplements.** There are some herbal supplements and natural remedies that sufferers of fibromyalgia have indicated have helped control their fibromyalgia symptoms. These include black cohosh, Echinacea, lavender, B vitamins, milk thistle, and cayenne pepper. These supplements have very little modern research showing their effectiveness in treating fibromyalgia symptoms. Talk to your doctor or herbalist before trying any of these supplements for your fibromyalgia symptoms.

Knowing which natural supplement or herb will be beneficial in controlling your fibromyalgia symptoms can be difficult. There can be drug-supplement interactions that only your doctor, a pharmacist, or a qualified herbalist knows about.

Most herbal remedies are not recommended for use by pregnant women, breastfeeding women, those with weakened immune systems, children, or the elderly—in part, because there are so few research studies done on the use of supplements in these populations of people.

Herbal remedies are not completely benign and can have serious interactions with anti-inflammatory medications or other medications used for pain. Others can result in an upset stomach if taken in excessive doses. Still others can result in excessive sedation or can thin your blood when taken for fibromyalgia symptoms. In such cases, your doctor or pharmacist can be valuable resources as you navigate your way through taking natural supplements for the management of your fibromyalgia.

Diet

Finding foods that can help your fibromyalgia may just be a matter of trial and error. There are very few research studies on the effect of diet on this chronic disease, leaving those with fibromyalgia to see which foods tend to make them feel better and those foods that make their symptoms worse. There are some general trends, however, in foods that are felt to impact fibromyalgia in positive or negative ways.

Let's look at what we do know about your diet and fibromyalgia to give you some idea of where to start in using diet to regulate your symptoms.

- **Try foods high in vitamin D.** Foods with vitamin D include fortified dairy products that also contain calcium for good bone health. Many people are deficient in vitamin D because they use sunscreen or live in higher latitudes where vitamin D can't be gotten from sunshine. Deficiencies of vitamin D have been known to cause symptoms similar to fibromyalgia. If you have fibromyalgia, you should be checked for vitamin D deficiency and load up on foods high in vitamin D if the levels return as low. Vitamin D deficiency has also been linked to having an insensitivity to the taking 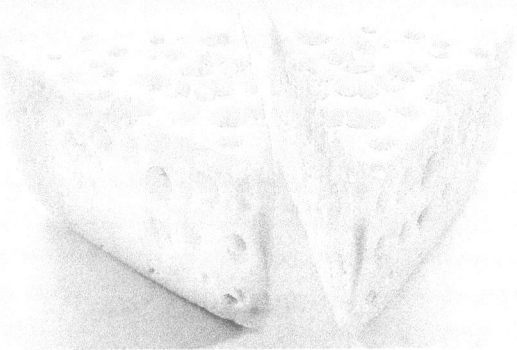 of pain relieving medication. If you don't think you can get enough vitamin D in your diet alone, try taking vitamin D supplements, especially during the winter when vitamin D from the sun is harder to come by.

- **Eat an anti-inflammatory diet.** Eating foods that prevent inflammation in the body helps to lessen pain. Two good anti-inflammatory diets are the Mediterranean diet and the Zone diet. In general, an anti-inflammatory diet includes the following:

  - Avoiding trans and saturated fats that come from processed foods and fatty meats.
  - Eating lots of different whole fruits and vegetables.
  - High intake of omega 3 fatty acids, found in fish, and walnuts.

- Reducing the intake of pasta, white rice, and refined carbohydrates.
- Eating lean protein sources, such as chicken and turkey.
- Reducing the intake of red meat and high fat dairy products.
- Eliminating processed foods and junk food.
- Adding spices such as ginger, garlic and curry for their anti-inflammatory benefits.

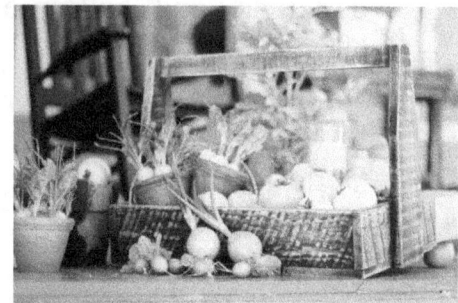

- **Stay away from food additives.** Many foods contain additives like aspartame and MSG (monosodium glutamate) that activate your brain's neurons, making them more sensitive to pain. Small studies have been done on people with fibromyalgia who eliminated these food additives from their diet and experienced a reduction in their fibromyalgia symptoms. Avoiding these additives cannot hurt you in the slightest and may make your symptoms much less noticeable.

- **Eat more fish.** Fish that are high in omega 3 fatty acids, such as salmon and tuna, have been found to reduce the body's level of inflammation and are known to be preventative against heart disease. One recent study also indicated that a diet high in omega 3 fatty acids reduced the symptoms of painful joints and morning stiffness in patients who did not have fibromyalgia. While fibromyalgia patients were not included in the study, it did include patients who had irritable bowel syndrome and rheumatoid arthritis, which are found along with patients who have fibromyalgia. It makes sense that omega 3 fatty acids may help fibromyalgia patients as well. Omega 3 fatty acids are found in more foods other than fish. You can find these healthful fatty acids in flaxseeds and walnuts as well.

- **Stay away from caffeine.** Caffeine is known to cause you to be jittery and can interfere with sleep, something that fibromyalgia patients struggle with and get too little of. While it may be tempting to use caffeine to combat daytime fatigue seen in fibromyalgia, this may backfire on you so that you lose sleep at night when you really need it. The "high" of caffeine also comes with a "crash" so you may be setting yourself up for more fatigue than you bargained for. Try drinking green tea instead, which has less caffeine in it and is high in antioxidants.

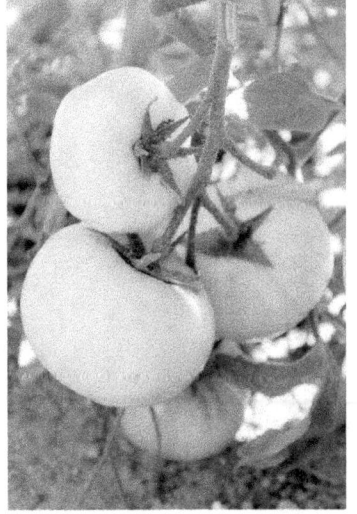

- **Eat more vegetables.** Vegetables are high in antioxidants, which combat oxidative stress. Some research experts believe that high amounts of oxygen free radicals contribute to many of the symptoms seen in fibromyalgia. By eating fruits and vegetables, you can get the anti-oxidant power to fight of oxygen free radicals along with high amounts of healthful vitamins. A raw, vegan diet would be ideal but if you can't tolerate such a strict diet, just incorporate as many colorful vegetables in your diet as you can.

Alternative Medicine

Alternative medicine offers viable, natural therapies that may either replace or complement conventional medical care to bring pain relief, and improve quality of life.

There are many of such therapies used successfully by those who suffer from Fibromyalgia and include but are not limited to:

- Acupuncture
- Herbalism
- Nutrition Therapy
- Massage
- Muscle Relaxation Therapy
- Reflexology
- Hydrotherapy
- Positive Affirmations
- Aromatherapy and Essential Oils
- Various Relaxation Methods
- Gentle Stretching Exercises

Keeping an open mind and looking into these various therapies may improve your quality of life, and diminish your pain. A holistic medicine practitioner can help you access and evaluate all these treatment methods as best suited for your specific case.

Living With Chronic Pain

Chronic pain can be very debilitating and affects all aspects of a person's life. Living with chronic pain is a 24/7 experience affecting the person throughout the day and well into the night. The pain alone is enough to limit one's life experiences; those with fibromyalgia have more than just chronic pain to deal with. They deal with emotional and mental symptoms as well as other physical symptoms that make chronic pain only part of what a person with fibromyalgia has to go through.

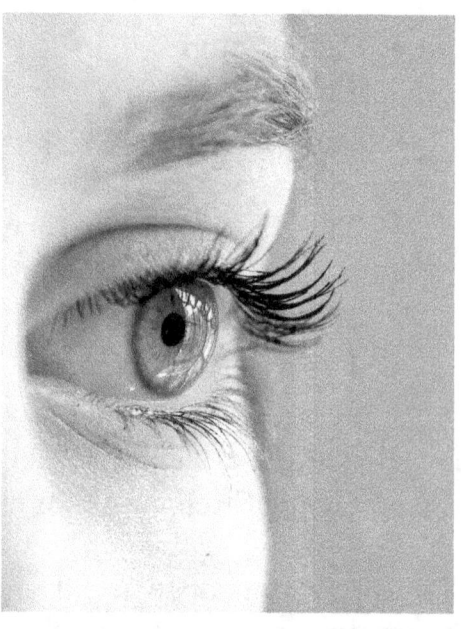

Unfortunately, modern science has little to offer those dealing with chronic pain. Even strong narcotic medications do little to controlling the symptoms and have side effects that make taking them difficult to live through, not to mention the very real addiction risks.

Some relief can be found by making an appointment with a reputable pain clinic. They deal with fibromyalgia patients all the time and have the skills it takes to both diagnose and treat your pain without having to resort to strong drugs or face a life of disability. While chronic pain is just a part of what goes into the diagnosis of fibromyalgia, treating the pain can go a long way in improving the quality of life of those who suffer from the disease.

Common Frustrations Of Sufferers

People with fibromyalgia did not ask to be sick and many led active lives before being struck down with the disease. This can lead to frustration, anxiety, and depression when you no longer can do the things your body allowed you to do in the past.

Lying in bed or on the couch all day can be devastating and can affect one's ability to lead a fruitful life. It can mean the difference between being a productive member of society to becoming an invalid. Many patients with fibromyalgia feel betrayed by their bodies and helpless to do anything about their symptoms. It doesn't help when doctors fail to properly diagnose the condition and have little in the way to offer those who suffer from fibromyalgia in 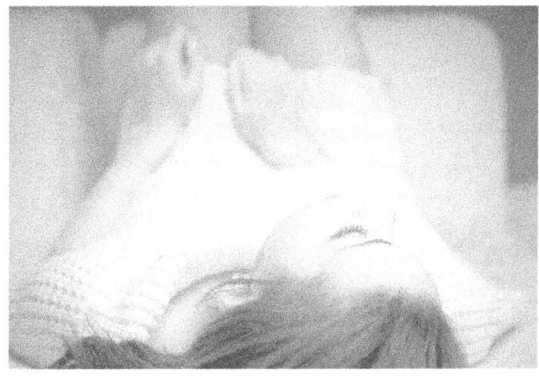 the way of treatments for the disease.

Many people with fibromyalgia are labeled as "complainers" or people who can't handle their emotions by those who have no understanding of the disease or doubt its validity. They are written off as being lazy or people who are just looking for narcotic pain relief for symptoms that can't be proven by medical science.

Fibromyalgia is a real disease that causes real disability in millions of people throughout the world. Perhaps it helps to know that through the treatments described above that many with fibromyalgia get some relief of their symptoms without having to resort to addictive medications.

There is a lot of research out there on fibromyalgia, including those looking into its origin and treatments that might help cure the condition. More and more is being learned about with regard to the disease every day. In the meantime, there are therapies that can help and they should be tried rather than giving into the pain and disability of the condition.

Support groups are highly recommended as surrounding yourself with like-minded who really understand your plight can be the best therapy for mind, body and spirit.

20 Tips For Dealing With Fibromyalgia

- Seek out medical professionals who really understand Fibromyalgia, and that you feel meet your needs and provide you with the time you need in each appointment.
- Do your own research into treatments and research scientific findings of this disease.
- Work to accept your body as it is, and be realistic of your present abilities.
- Never push yourself beyond what you are physically capable of, do what you can and appreciate those abilities.
- Seek out and try every possible treatment option, especially the natural methods found in alternative medicine. Remember that any type of therapy that can improve quality of life and symptoms should be investigated and given a chance to work.

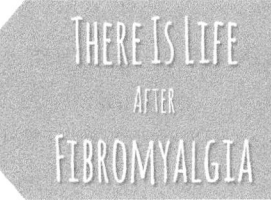

- Set realistic goals so you can feel accomplished and good about yourself, instead of trying to reach unattainable feats that can lead to loss of confidence, depression, and anxiety.
- Surround yourself with supportive, positive, and understanding people who give you the emotional support you need.
- Be vigilant about your mental health, if you feel yourself slipping into depression, which is common

among patients; seek help from a qualified professional.

- Talk, talk and talk some more. Express all your feelings, especially your anger, frustrations, anxiety, and fears to trusted sources.
- Cry when you need to. Crying is a great release of feelings.
- Attend support groups where you can get understanding and give some back to others.
- Eliminate all possible sources of stress and partake in stress reducing activities. Aromatherapy, good sleep, low stress work, happy relationships, and many other actions can help reduce stress to improve the outlook of your condition and quality of life.
- Take a moment to mourn your old life, and then take days to look forward to your new life.
- Rewrite your life. If you used to run marathons, it may be time to get to let that go, instead design an exercise plan you can achieve and stick with those goals. You might have to change jobs, or get more help with the kids than you used to, it's okay, making these changes is all part of the acceptance.
- Ask for help. Do not let pride stand in the way of getting help as you need it, no matter the circumstances.
- Look for the silver linings and practice positive thinking. Life presents us with harsh lessons and circumstances, but there is always a positive side, look for it and revel in it. For example, perhaps you have made a new special best friend in a support group that is one positive aspect of fibromyalgia.
- Revel in your strength, and resolve and see your coping ability as a positive aspect of this disease. Be proud that you are so resilient that you can handle

anything life throws at you.

- Stay away from negative people who doubt your symptoms and are not supportive, their negativity is like poison that can really damage your outlook, and wellness.
- Consider for a moment people who are blind and work full time and those who are deaf but married with children, there are also those in wheelchairs participating in Olympic Games and playing basketball. While it would be easy for people with such profound disabilities to lay down and give up, they don't, they live full lives and accept what is, and so can you.
- Consider and accept that you may not be as powerless as you may believe. While you may have lost power over some of your physical abilities, or perhaps how others view you, you absolutely have the power over how you view yourself.

Improving Your Quality Of Life

It is simply not true that those who suffer from fibromyalgia face a lifetime of pain and disability. Once the diagnosis is made and treatments begun, strides can be made in controlling each symptom of fibromyalgia as it comes along. Sometimes taking matters just one day at a time is enough to make things more manageable.

Fibromyalgia waxes and wanes so that there will be days where you can accomplish things you have been wanting to do. Therapies like exercise and anti-depressant therapy can cut through the fog of fibromyalgia so that not every day has to be a total washout.

Listen to your body and what it is telling you. Pace yourself according to your symptoms.

Know that, while there is not yet a cure for the disease, there are promising modalities that lessen the symptoms so that you can deal with the pain and go about as many daily activities as you can.

You are not alone!

Seek out a support group for those who suffer with fibromyalgia and other forms of chronic pain so that you can find ways that others have used to successfully manage their symptoms and find support and friendship with people who really understand.

Fibromyalgia does not have to mean you are at the end of a productive life. People with fibromyalgia find ways to be gainfully employed and carry on with successful relationships in spite of their pain and other symptoms.

By reading this guide, hopefully you have found some ideas you can use to improve the quality of your life even though you live with a difficult disease.

Stay well and take care!

The End

www.ingramcontent.com/pod-product-compliance
Lightning Source LLC
Chambersburg PA
CBHW070323290526
45791CB00003B/1234